THE ORIGINAL KETO COOKBOOK

LOSE WEIGHT WITH DELICIOUS AND HEALHTY
RECIPES INCL. 14 DAYS KETO DIET MEAL PREP PLAN

[1st Edition]

Kate Evans

Have you heard of the ketogenic, better known as keto, diet? As it seems to be all the rage right now, most people have heard of at least some variation, of the keto diet. Similar diets are banting, paleo, or even the Atkins diet. All of them revolve around the concept of a high intake of good fat and a low intake of carbohydrates. Carbohydrates, in this instance, means things like white bread, pasta, sugary drinks, and foods. Yes, things we all indulge in, sometimes on a daily basis. The plan behind eating more good fats is to get more calories from the proteins than the carbs. Reducing your daily carb intake to less than 50gr will tell your body it's running out of glucose (blood sugar) for your required energy. So your body then starts to look for an alternative source to make energy: proteins and fats. Once your body starts burning fats, you have reached a stage called ketosis, and you will start to lose weight. What a wonderful thought! And doesn't it sound so easy?

Benefits of following the Keto diet

While keto most definitely has benefits for people wanting to lose weight, it also has significant benefits for people suffering from various illnesses. A sad reality of today's unhealthy lifestyles is an increase in people getting Type 2 diabetes. A few studies have shown that some people living with type 2 diabetes have actually reversed its effects when they followed the keto diet. This is because the food you eat reduces your blood sugar levels naturally. If you've been diagnosed with Type 2 diabetes, the keto diet may just be the answer for you. If we can reduce the number of pills we take a day, just by eating the right foods, isn't that what we should aim for? Another illness that keto helps with is epilepsy. This diet was first introduced in the early 1900s aimed at children who have epilepsy, although the diet was probably called something else. The results were so good that the keto lifestyle is being encouraged to all people living with epilepsy around the world. A lot of them have also reported using fewer pharmaceutical drugs too. Again, reducing our pill intake!

Another fabulous benefit is finding you can focus and concentrate more effectively. The alternative fuel source that keto creates from burning your fat is called ketones. These ketones are an amazing fuel source for your brain. Reducing your carb intake also reduces blood sugar spikes, which, when combined with the ketones, allows you to stay alert for longer. This benefit alone has encouraged a lot of professionals in high-pressure jobs to follow the keto diet.

Do you have acne? Studies still need to understand this more, but there is definite evidence that following keto has some advantages in diminishing acne. It is a well-known fact that eating too much fast foods can have an effect on your skin, but acne can also be a result of hormone imbalances. Correcting your eating habits by following the keto diet will have an all-round positive reaction.

Have you noticed that sometimes you will eat a meal and within two hours, maybe even less, you're hungry again? This is because whatever you ate is probably a high glycemic index meal. You get an initial sugar spike which boosts your energy, but you quickly burn through that energy, making you feel hungry long before your next meal. Keto foods are low-gi, which digests slower and therefore, doesn't spike your blood sugar levels. So your meal will satisfy you, and you can go for longer periods without thinking about your next meal, or snacking on something bad.

As you now know, the keto diet aims at getting you to eat more protein and good fats, hence the 'high fat - low carb' nickname. So it might seem a little weird that this can have heart health benefits, seeing as doctors are always saying cut out all that red meat. But the fact is, it does! Studies still need to examine this phenomenon, but it seems that because the keto diet lowers your insulin levels, your body stops creating cholesterol, which we know clogs arteries. This has a direct benefit on heart health and those who suffer from high blood pressure, heart failure and the like. Of course, high blood pressure is often associated with being overweight too, so as you shed those pounds, have your doctor check out your heart and see if still need to take those blood pressure pills.

Those fad diets where you have to weigh your portions or count the calories are so incredibly time-consuming and not to mention, annoying. Most people on those kinds of diets give up after a week because it's just too much work, and it takes ages to see any noticeable results. Losing weight and getting healthier should be effortless and enjoyable, not a chore. Keto does require a mindset change, but because you will see results quickly, you'll be encouraged and therefore will be more likely to continue on the lifestyle. It is a lifestyle change and a drastic one at that. If you're serious about losing the extra pounds, whether its doctor ordered or just to fit into last season's jeans, you won't go wrong following keto. Just make sure you are in the right mindset and know the foods you're allowed and those you have to toss out of your life. There is a little bit of counting involved, but it more relates to learning to read labels than actual counting. The typical amounts you should be eating per day are 65% fats, 25% proteins, and 10% carbs. So when you pick up something interesting at the store, be sure to look at the nutritional facts first. You will actually be shocked at the high levels of carbs and processed sugars in some foods that are supposed to be healthy for you!

Some tips to get you started

The first week is always the hardest. It's going to send your body into shock, and it might be easier if you had someone to do it with you, like a family member or good friend. Teamwork makes the dream work, right? Mentally getting through is half the battle won and when you're down, your friend and motivate you with a delicious keto-friendly dessert (recipes in here!), or vice versa.

Getting into the keto mindset will help if you're strict with yourself in the first week. Try to keep your daily carb intake under 20 grams. As you progress and learn to know which foods work with you, you can increase or decrease. Just remember that on the whole, your carb intake must be around 10% per day.

WATER! WATER! WATER! This stuff, even if you're not on a diet, is your best friend! Drink as much water as possible to flush out everything from your system. Yes, the bathroom will become the room you spend a lot of time in, but it will be worth it. Don't swop other drinks like tea and coffee for your water intake either. That's cheating. And by all means, if you don't like tap water, get those bottles of spring water chilling in the fridge.

Fruits are not your friend on the other hand. Yes, some fruits you can eat, but it's mainly the ones from the berry family that you can. Most fruits are not allowed because they have a high amount of carbs.

Here's one that every dieter dreads: exercise. You don't have to join a gym and have to feel like all the gorgeous gym-bunnies are staring at you. All that's required is some form of light exercise to get your heart rate going. A walk around the block or the park should suffice. And walking with a friend will make it easier and quicker. If we're truly honest with ourselves, sitting around all day is doing nothing for us. If you have a busy schedule, go for a walk during your lunch or even as a family after dinner. Taking the dog for a walk is also a good excuse to get out and about.

There will be days when you're just "not feeling it". Set goals for yourself and be realistic about them. Also, remember that everyone's keto journey is different, so don't compare yourself to other keto users' experiences. Find out what works for you and keep at it, the results will come.

The start of your keto journey begins with going through your cupboards. Yes, and those secret stashes! If you're sitting around and suddenly remember there's a chocolate bar somewhere, your brain will focus on that and will drive you nuts. GET RID OF IT! There will be days when you're craving, and one small chocolate bar now and again won't hurt. But make them a prize for yourself. Don't have it waiting in your cupboard. Make sure you reach a goal and then go out and buy it to enjoy.

Temptations come in all forms, and sure you can get rid of them from your home, but what about your friend's birthday at that fancy restaurant next week? Don't be scared to go and eat out. Once you learn all the foods you can and can't have, you can go through the menu and select whatever you want, just ask the waiter if it's possible to swap some items out. For example, swap out the fries for a portion of veg. Have a burger but without the buns. Most restaurants are happy to oblige, and another bonus is that some restaurants have keto-friendly options.

Here is a brief overview of the foods you can and can't eat. Getting to know them is vital to help you along your way, especially when you're at a restaurant or getting your groceries.

The Permitted List

- Vegetables: Leafy green veg and all veg that grows above ground are allowed. Kale, lettuce, broccoli, tomatoes, etc.

- High-fat dairy: Whole milk, fresh cream, full-fat cheese.

- Meat: All the meats are permitted! Beef, pork, lamb, chicken, etc.

- Berries: Strawberries, blueberries, avocados (Yes, it's a berry!), raspberries.

- Sugar alternatives are quite vast nowadays, with Erythritol, stevia, xylitol and monk fruit, to name a few. You might have seen xylitol in chewing gum and stevia in soft drinks. These have become alternatives to the sweeteners with aspartame, which can be a health hazard. Just a side note about xylitol, especially if you have pets: it's lethal for them.

- Condiments aren't all banned either, so you can spice up that steak! Stick to salt, pepper, herbs, and spices though.

- Other good fats include olive oil, coconut oil, high-fat salad dressings, butter, and nut butter.

- Seeds and nuts make an excellent snack or a dessert topping — cashews, macadamias, chia seeds, etc.

The Banned List

- High sugar content foods are obviously not allowed. Cakes, chocolate bars, ice cream, soda, even 100% fruit juice has too much sugar and carbs!

- We already mentioned fruit as being a no-no, due to the high natural carbs and sugars in them.

- Wheat products are banned, so anything like bread, cereals, pasta, and rice must be eliminated from your grocery cupboard. A simple way to remember this is to check if it was made with white flour. If the answer is yes, put it back on the shelf.

- Legumes and beans. This includes peas, chickpeas, anything with the name bean in it and peanuts. Peanuts are not a nut like some people think, they are actually a legume.

- Any veg that grows underground like potatoes and carrots. Sadly, they have too many carbs.

- Watch out for sauces and condiments. Yes there some that are allowed, but things like ketchup and bbq sauce often have high sugar content and therefore are not allowed.

- Alcohol also has too many carbs, so rather go for that glass of water.

- All cooking oils, margarine, and mayonnaises are banned, as they only contain bad fats.

- Do not even look at the diet foods! Just have a look at the labels, and you will see the high amounts of processed sugars and carbs! They will not be a help to you in any way.

With these lists, you may be thinking what on earth can I eat? Well, with this book, you will be getting some incredibly delicious recipes, that you can chop and change as you get used to the keto lifestyle. If you find you're getting hungry before your next meal, snack on some nuts or even a spoonful of nut butter. You can even increase your meals from 3 to 5 smaller portions a day. It all depends on you and finding your balance.

RECIPES

Serves: 1

kCal: 445 |Carbs: 6.34g |Fat: 38.16g | Protein: 10.45g

INGREDIENTS

- 2 tablespoons / 28gr grounds flaxseed
- 1 tablespoon / 14gr almond meal
- ½ teaspoon / 2.5gr vanilla powder
- 1 tablespoon / 14gr of desiccated coconut
- ½ teaspoon / 2.5gr cinnamon
- ⅓ cup / 80ml coconut milk
- ½ cup / 120ml of almond milk
- ¼ cup / 85gr of mixed berries
- 1 teaspoon / 5gr of dried pumpkin seeds

DIRECTIONS

1. Preheat a saucepan on the stove
2. Keep the berries and pumpkins seeds aside and add the rest to the saucepan
3. Stir the mixture until it resembles oatmeal/porridge
4. Pour into a bowl, add the berries and seeds and serve

Serves: 5

kCal: 412 | Carbs: 2.26g | Fat: 31.66g | Protein: 28.21g

INGREDIENTS

- 10 large eggs
- Salt
- Pepper

- 1½ cups / 510gr of grated cheddar
- 5 slices of cooked bacon
- 5 cooked breakfast sausage patties

DIRECTIONS

1. Preheat a non-stick skillet onmedium-high
2. Whisk two of the eggs in a bowl
3. Once the skillet is hot, lower the heat to medium-low and add the whisked eggs
4. Sprinkle some salt and pepper onto the eggs
5. Using a lid, cover the egg mixture and cook until almost done all the way through
6. Sprinkle some cheese, add a strip of bacon and half of a patty onto the egg
7. Carefully roll up the egg like a wrap. It can be fiddly, so take it slowly
8. Repeat the steps for 4 more wraps to end up with 5 and serve

Serves: 1

kCal: 515 | Carbs: 4.17g | Fat: 39.58g | Protein: 21.34g

INGREDIENTS

- 3 large eggs
- 2 teaspoons / 10ml heavy cream
- 3oz / 85gr of sliced mushrooms
- 1 teaspoon / 5ml of olive oil
- 2oz / 56gr goats cheese, crumbled
- Spike seasoning to taste
- For some optional garnish, you can have some green onions

DIRECTIONS

1. In a frying pan, heat the oil and fry mushrooms until they are soft.
2. In a mixing bowl whisk together the eggs, cream and Spike seasoning.
3. Take the cooked mushrooms out of the pan and set aside.
4. Add the egg mix to the pan and cook for 2 – 3 mins.
5. As the egg mixture begins to set, add the mushrooms and goats cheese.
6. Very carefully fold the egg mixture over to form the omelet.
7. Cook until the cheese begins to melt.
8. Serve and garnish if desired.

Serves: 1

kCal: 333 | Carbs: 4.28g | Fat: 22.66g | Protein: 25.59g

INGREDIENTS

- 3 large eggs, separated
- 4 tablespoons / 57gr of grated mozzarella cheese
- 1 teaspoon / 5gr Italian herb blend
- 2 large sliced black olives
- 4 large mild pepper rings
- 1 tablespoon / 15gr of diced red bell pepper
- 1 tablespoon / 15gr of tomato sauce

DIRECTIONS

1. Spray 2 microwave-safe ramekin-sized bowls with cooking spray
2. Add 1 tablespoon of the cheese and herbs to each bowl
3. In a mixing bowl, beat the egg whites until frothy and add to the ramekins
4. Microwave until the whites are cooked, should be about 1 – 2 mins and then allow to cool
5. Beat the egg yolks and scramble them lightly in a frying pan
6. Fold in the olives and peppers into the scrambled eggs
7. Remove from the heat
8. Add some tomato sauce to your "pizza bases" in the ramekins
9. Add the scrambled egg mix and the remaining cheese to the "pizza bases"
10. Cook for another 20 secs, until the cheese has melted
11. Serve hot

Serves: 2

kCal: 481 | Carbs: 1.28g | Fat: 37.97g | Protein: 31.76g

INGREDIENTS

- ◆ 4oz / 113gr of sausage
- ◆ 2oz / 57gr of pepper jack cheese
- ◆ 4 slices of bacon
- ◆ 2 large eggs
- ◆ 1 tablespoon / 4.71gr of butter
- ◆ 1 tablespoon / 7gr of PB Fit Powder (available online and in health stores)
- ◆ Salt
- ◆ Pepper

DIRECTIONS

1. Heat the oven to 400°F / 205°C and cook your bacon for 20 to 25 mins
2. Mix the PB Fit powder with the butter and set aside.
3. With your sausage, form burger patties and cook on both sides. Add the cheese on top, allow to melt and take out the pan
4. Fry the eggs as desired
5. Assemble your burgers as desired and serve

Serves: 1

kCal: 698 | Carbs: 3.09g | Fat: 54.95g | Protein: 41.91g

INGREDIENTS

- The Pancake
- 0.75oz / 21gr of pork rinds
- 1 tablespoon / 6gr almond flour
- 1 large egg, beaten
- 1 tablespoon / 15ml of heavy cream
- ¼ teaspoon/ 2ml of vanilla extract

- 2 tablespoons / 30ml of sugar-free maple syrup
- The Filling
- 2oz / 57gr of sausage
- 1 slice of cheddar
- 1 large egg

DIRECTIONS

1. Form the sausage into a patty shape with the help of a ring mold, preferably silicone

2. Cook in a pan over a medium heat until done

3. Set aside on some foil

4. Grind the pork rinds until they are a powder and mix with all the pancake Ingredients to form a batter

5. Place the ring mold back into the pan and fill halfway with the batter

6. Cook on one side until brown, remove mold, flip and cook the other side.

7. Repeat until you have 2 pancakes

8. Using the ring mold again scramble your last egg for the filling

9. Assemble your Pancake Sandwich and serve

Serves: 12

kCal: 157.17 | Carbs: 1.35g | Fat: 12.28g | Protein: 9.75g

INGREDIENTS

- 4oz / 117gr of cheddar cheese
- 3oz / 85gr of cream cheese
- 4 medium jalapeno peppers, de-seeded and chopped
- 12 bacon strips
- 8 large eggs
- ½ teaspoon / 2.5gr garlic powder
- ½ teaspoon 2.5gr of onion powder
- Salt
- Pepper

DIRECTIONS

1. Heat the oven to 374°F / 190°C

2. Fry your bacon until its semi-crisp. Save the bacon grease for the next step

3. Using a mixer, mix together the eggs, bacon grease, cream cheese, garlic and onion powders, and 3 of the peppers (save 1 for toppings)

4. Grease a muffin tin well, and place the semi-cooked bacon around the edges of the wells so that it will form the sides of a cup

5. Pour into the wells, the egg mixture, but do not overfill them. Two-thirds should be ample, as they rise quite a bit

6. Add the cheddar cheese and the remaining jalapeno on top

7. Bake for 20 to 25 mins, allow to cool then serve

Serves: 4

kCal: 322.35 | Carbs: 3.1g | Fat: 22.15g | Protein: 24.23g

INGREDIENTS

- ◆ 8 large eggs
- ◆ 5oz / 142gr bacon slices
- ◆ 12 cherry tomatoes (can use more if desired)
- ◆ ¼ cup / 6½gr fresh parsley, chopped

DIRECTIONS

1. Over a medium heat, fry the bacon until crispy
2. Once done, plate the bacon, but leave the bacon grease in the pan
3. Cook the eggs in the bacon grease however you want (fried, scrambled, etc.)
4. Add the eggs to the plate
5. Roast the tomatoes in the same pan, for a few mins
6. Add to the plate, garnish with the parsley and serve

Serves: 5

kCal: 406.4 | Carbs: 3.58g | Fat: 35.85g | Protein: 19.63g

INGREDIENTS

- ◆ 3 tablespoons / 44ml olive oil
- ◆ ½ of a medium-sized onion, diced
- ◆ 1½ teaspoons / 7.5gr of minced garlic
- ◆ 6oz / 170gr of ham steak, cubed and cooked
- ◆ 1 tablespoon / 14gr of butter for greasing
- ◆ 6 large eggs
- ◆ 1 cup / 235gr ofgrated cheddar
- ◆ ½ cup / 118ml heavy cream
- ◆ 2 tablespoons / 6.5gr of fresh chives, chopped
- ◆ ½ teaspoon / 2.5gr of salt
- ◆ ½ teaspoon / 1.2gr of black pepper

DIRECTIONS

1. Heat the oven to 400°F / 205°C
2. In a pan, heat the olive oil and add the onions, cook until soft.
3. Add the garlic and cook until brown
4. In a mixing bowl, add all the remaining Ingredients, and the cooked onions and garlic, and mix together well.
5. Grease 5 ramekins with the butter
6. Divide the mixture equally amongst the ramekins
7. Bake for 20mins
8. Let cool slightly and then serve warm

Serves: 8

kCal: 206.81 | Carbs: 3.53g | Fat: 18.5g | Protein: 6.6g

INGREDIENTS

- 1½ cups / 144gr of almond flour
- 2 tablespoons/ 9gr of coconut flour
- 1 tablespoon / 2.5gr of psyllium husk
- ½ teaspoon / 2.5gr of baking powder
- ¼ teaspoon / 1.2gr of baking soda

- 1 tablespoon / 9gr of poppy seeds
- 4 tablespoons / 57gr of butter
- ¼ cup / 50gr of erythritol
- 2 large eggs
- ½ lemon, juice and zest
- 2 tablespoons / 25gr of erythritol for sprinkling

DIRECTIONS

1. Heat the oven to 350°F / 180°C

2. Line a baking sheet with parchment paper

3. In a large mixing bowl, combine the almond flour, coconut flour, psyllium husk, baking powder, and baking soda

4. Add in the poppy seeds and mix until well combined

5. Cut the butter into the dry mixture, continue mixing until a dough forms

6. In another bowl, whisk the eggs and erythritol together until frothy

7. Zest the lemon onto a plate, add the sprinkling erythritol to the zest

8. Using a fork, mash the zest and the erythritol together, then set aside to dry

9. Cut the lemon in half and squeeze the juice into the egg mixture, be careful not to let any seeds escape the lemon, the pulp is okay though

10. Pour the egg mixture into the dough and combine well

11. Place the dough onto the parchment paper and shape into adome

12. Score the dough into 8 triangles

13. Bake for 20 mins

14. Take out the over, cut the 8 triangles and separate

15. Sprinkle with the lemon sugar and bake for another 10 mins

Serves: 11

kCal: 231.36 | Carbs: 1.96g | Fat: 21.9g | Protein: 5.03g

INGREDIENTS

- 1 cup / 96gr almond flour
- ½ cup / 48gr golden flaxseed
- ¾ cup / 90gr pecan halves
- ½ cup / 105gr coconut oil
- 2 large eggs
- ¼ cup / 50gr erythritol
- 2 teaspoons / 10ml maple extract
- 1 teaspoon / 5ml vanilla extract
- ½ teaspoon / 2.5gr baking soda
- ½ teaspoon / 2.5ml apple cider vinegar
- ¼ teaspoon / 1.2ml liquid stevia

DIRECTIONS

1. Preheat the oven to 325°F / 160°C
2. Chop the pecans finely, preferably with a food processor. Put 2/3rds of the pecans in a large mixing bowl and set the remaining 1/3rd aside
3. In a separate mixing bowl, combine all the wet Ingredients
4. Add the remaining dry Ingredients to the pecans in the mixing bowl and combine
5. Add the dry and wet mixtures together well
6. Divide the batter equally into 11 muffin/cupcake liners in a muffin/cupcake baking tray
7. Sprinkle the left over pecans over the muffins and bake for 25 – 30 mins

Serves: 12

kCal: 195.5 | Carbs: 3.49g | Fat: 17.47g | Protein: 5.49g

INGREDIENTS

- ◆ 1⅓ cup / 164gr coconut flour (sifted)
- ◆ 3 teaspoons / 14gr baking powder
- ◆ 1 teaspoon / 67gr dried ground sage
- ◆ ½ teaspoon / 2.5gr salt
- ◆ ¼ teaspoon / 0.85gr garlic powder
- ◆ 2 cups / 473ml canned coconut milk
- ◆ ½ cup / 118ml water
- ◆ 3 tablespoons / 45ml melted coconut oil
- ◆ 1 cup / 235gr grated cheddar

DIRECTIONS

1. Heat your waffle iron to a medium heat
2. Whisk together the flour, baking powder, and seasonings
3. Add all the liquid Ingredients and mix together until it forms a stiff batter
4. Combine the cheese into the batter
5. Grease your waffle iron well
6. Scoop 1/3 cup of batter onto each waffle iron section
7. Close the iron and cook until steam rises and the iron opens without the waffle sticking
8. Repeat until all batter is used

Serves: 6

kCal: 424 | Carbs: 3.63g | Fat: 34.82g | Protein: 22.9g

INGREDIENTS

- 7 bacon slices
- 1 tablespoon / 15ml of olive oil
- 4 large mushroom caps
- 2 tablespoons / 5gr fresh parsley
- ½ cup / 13gr fresh basil, chopped
- 4oz / 113gr fresh mozzarella, cubed
- 2oz / 56gr hard goats cheese, grated
- 1 medium red bell pepper
- 8 large eggs
- ¼ cup / 118ml heavy cream
- ¼ cup / 35gr parmesan cheese, grated
- Salt
- Pepper

DIRECTIONS

1. Preheat oven to 350°F / 180°C

2. Roughly chop the basil, pepper, mushrooms, and bacon

3. Add olive oil to an oven-proof hot pan and wait for the first wisp of smoke. The moment you see it, add the bacon and cook until browned.

4. Add the pepper to the bacon and cook until soft

5. In a mixing bowl, add the parmesan cheese, cream, eggs, and pepper and whisk until combined

6. Once the peppers are done, add the mushrooms and stir well, allowing the mushrooms to soak in the fat

7. Add the basil, cook for a few seconds and then add the cubed mozzarella

8. Pour the egg mixture over everything and make sure everything is well combined

9. Sprinkle the grated goats cheese over everything

10. Put the oven-proof pan in the oven and bake for 6 – 8 mins

11. Then change to grill and grill for 4 – 6 mins

12. Take out the oven and carefully pry the edges away from the pan to make flipping easier

13. Flip onto a serving platter, slice and serve

Serves: 5

kCal: 211.4 | Carbs: 4.74g | Fat: 17.56g | Protein: 10.09g

INGREDIENTS

- 14oz / 397gr firm tofu
- 3 tablespoons /45ml avocado oil
- 2 tablespoons / 6.5gr diced yellow onion
- 1½ tablespoons / 28gr nutritional yeast
- ½ tablespoon / 2.5gr garlic powder
- ½ teaspoon / 2.5gr of turmeric
- ½ teaspoon / 2.6gr salt
- 1 cup / 340gr baby spinach
- 3grape tomatoes, diced
- 3oz / 88gr vegan cheddar

DIRECTIONS

1. Wrap your tofu in some paper towels and gently squeeze some of the water out
2. Place a skillet on a medium heat and add 1/3rd of the avocado oil. Sauté the onion in the oil until soft
3. Add the tofu to the skillet and crumble with a fork until it resembles scrambled egg
4. Drizzle the rest of the avo oil over it
5. Sprinkle the dry seasonings and stir to coat
6. Continue to cook thetofu, occasionally stirring, until most of the liquid has evaporated
7. Fold in the spinach, tomato, and cheese and cook until the cheese has melted
8. Serve hot
9. Can store leftovers in the fridge for up to 3 days

Serves: 16

kCal: 200.13 | Carbs: 2.6g | Fat: 18.83g | Protein: 5.59g

INGREDIENTS

- 3 large eggs
- ½ cup / 118ml olive oil
- 1 teaspoon / 5ml vanilla extract
- 2½ cups / 240gr almond flour
- 1½ cups / 300gr erythritol
- ½ teaspoon / 3gr salt
- 1½ teaspoons / 7gr baking powder
- ½ teaspoon / 1.2gr nutmeg
- 1 teaspoon / 2.6gr ground cinnamon
- ¼ teaspoon / 0.54gr ground ginger
- 1 cup / 150gr grated zucchini
- ½ cup / 60gr chopped walnuts

DIRECTIONS

1 Heat the oven to 350°F / 180°C

2. Whisk the eggs oil and vanilla extract and set aside

3. In another mixing bowl, mix the almond flour, erythritol, salt, baking powder, nutmeg, cinnamon and gingerand also set aside

4. Wrap the zucchini in paper towels and squeeze any excess water

5. Add the zucchini to the egg mixture and whisk together

6. Slowly add the dry Ingredients to the egg mixture and mix until fully combined

7. Spray some cooking spray onto a loaf tin (9x5) and add the dough mixture

8. Add the walnuts on top of the dough and gently press them into the dough

9. Bake for 60 – 70 mins or until the walnuts are browned

Serves: 4

kCal: 312.43 | Carbs: 3.12g | Fat: 22.11g | Protein: 24.91g

INGREDIENTS

- 8oz / 227gr smoked deli ham slices
- 8 slices of Swiss cheese
- 16 slices dill pickles
- 3 tablespoons / 45ml of Italian dressing
- ¼ tablespoon / 7.5ml of Italian seasoning

DIRECTIONS

1. Preheat your oven to 375°F / 190°C
2. Layer the ham across the bottom of a casserole dish
3. Add a layer of Swiss cheese on top of the ham
4. Add a layer of the dill pickles, dressing, and seasonings
5. Bake for 10 – 15 mins until the cheese has melted

Serves: 6

kCal: 169.13 | Carbs: 2.53g | Fat: 14.52g | Protein: 3.27g

INGREDIENTS

- 3 mediumavocados, halved, remove stone
- 1½ oz / 50gr chopped mushrooms
- 1 medium chopped green onion
- 10 chopped cherry tomatoes
- 1oz / 44grgoats cheese, crumbled
- 1 tablespoon / 15ml olive oil
- 1 tablespoon / 15ml liquid smoke
- ½ teaspoon / 2½gr paprika
- 3 tablespoons / 45ml balsamic vinegar

DIRECTIONS

1. Heat a frying panto a medium temperature
2. In a mixing bowl, add mushrooms, tomatoes, and onions
3. Heat the olive oil, liquid smoke, and paprika in the pan
4. To the pan add the cheese, and sauté until brown
5. Take off the heat and add the cheese mixture to the mixing bowl and mix well
6. Scoop out a bit of the avo to make it into a bowl
7. Add the mixture to the "bowl" and top off with a bit of scooped avo
8. Drizzle a ½ teaspoon of balsamic over each bowl and serve

Serves: 6

kCal: 388.37 | Carbs: 6.5g | Fat: 32.47g | Protein: 15.8g

INGREDIENTS

- 3/4lb / 340gr of ground beef
- 1 teaspoon / 5gr of ground cumin
- ½ teaspoon / 1.3gr of chili powder
- 1 teaspoon / ½gr dried parsley
- 1 teaspoon / 3gr of garlic powder

- 8oz / 227gr of chopped romaine lettuce
- 9oz / 255gr of chopped iceberg lettuce
- 2 small chopped red tomatoes
- 1½ cups / 180grmozzarella, grated
- 1 medium avocado, chopped
- 1 cup / 120gr of sour cream

DIRECTIONS

1. Add your beef, herbs, and spices to a non-stick frying pan, and cook on a medium heat
2. Once done, remove from the heat, drain the beef and set aside to cool
3. In a salad bowl, add all the lettuce, tomatoes, cheese and avo and mix well
4. Add the beef and sour cream on top, combine and serve

Serves: 5

kCal: 206.4 | Carbs: 4.33g | Fat: 14.59g | Protein: 11.55g

INGREDIENTS

- ◆ 2 medium zucchinis
- ◆ 8 slices of cooked bacon
- ◆ 1 cup / 200gr of feta cheese, cubed
- ◆ 1 cup / 200gr ofcherry tomatoes, chopped
- ◆ 4 tablespoons / 60ml balsamic vinegar

DIRECTIONS

1. Using a peeler or grater, slice the zucchinis long-ways into ribbons
2. Add the ribbons to a salad bowl, top off with the tomatoes, bacon, and cheese
3. Drizzle with the balsamic, toss and serve

Serves: 6

kCal: 512.17 | Carbs: 7.62g | Fat: 41.7g | Protein: 24.93g

INGREDIENTS

- ¾ cup / 96gr almond flour
- 2 cups / 450gr grated skim mozzarella
- 6 jumbo all-beef hot dogs
- ½ cup / 100gr fresh pineapple chunks
- 6 slices ham, diced
- 6 slices bacon, chopped
- 6 tablespoons / 85gr sarayo

DIRECTIONS

1. Preheat your oven to 350°F / 180°C
2. Place a non-stick pan over a medium heat
3. Melt the mozzarella and stir in the almond flour until a dough forms
4. Place the dough between two sheets of parchment and roll until flat
5. You can use a pot lid or a 6" bowl to cut out 6 circles
6. Prepare a baking sheet with some parchment paper and lay out the circles.
7. Bake for 10 mins
8. Warm up your dogs however you like, place in the middle of the bread circles and wrap
9. Top with pineapple, ham, bacon and serve

Serves: 4

kCal: 342.53 | Carbs: 1.68g | Fat: 14.8g | Protein: 47.6g

INGREDIENTS

- 24oz / 680gr jar of pickles
- 8 medium chicken breast tenders / fillets
- 2 scoops unflavored 100% whey protein powder
- ¼ cup / 22.5gr Parmesan, grated
- Salt
- Pepper
- 1 teaspoon / 2.5gr paprika
- 2 large eggs
- 2 tablespoons/ 30ml avocado oil

DIRECTIONS

1. Take the pickles out of the jar
2. Add the chicken pieces to a Ziploc bag and add the pickle juice
3. Place in the fridge and allow to marinate for one hour
4. In a mixing bowl, mix the cheese, protein powder, salt, pepper, and paprika
5. Beat the eggs in another bowl
6. Over a medium-high heat, preheat a skillet and add the avocado oil, allow it to heat up while you bread the chicken
7. Dip the chicken into the egg and then coat with the bread mixture
8. Fry them until they are golden brown and fully cooked through

Serves: 2

kCal: 537.55 | Carbs: 11.1g | Fat: 45.85g | Protein: 19.35g

INGREDIENTS

- The salad
- 1¼ cups / 280gr diced pumpkin
- 1 tablespoon / 15ml olive oil
- 1 teaspoon / 2.5gr paprika
- Salt
- 1 tablespoon / 5gr butter
- 4oz / 114gr halloumi, cubed
- 3 tablespoons / 15.6gr flaked almonds

- 6 cups / 200gr watercress
- ½ medium avocado, sliced
- The dressing
- 1 tablespoon / 15gr tahini
- 1 tablespoon / 15ml olive oil
- 1 tablespoon / 15ml lemon juice
- ⅛ teaspoon / 0.75gr salt
- ⅛ teaspoon / 0.61ml apple cider vinegar

DIRECTIONS

1. Preheat the oven to 400°F / 205°C

2. Mix together the diced pumpkin, olive oil, paprika, and salt, then spread it out evenly on a baking tray and roast for 15-20 mins, until it starts to brown and soften

3. In a non-stick pan melt the butter over a medium heat and fry the halloumi for 10-15 mins, stirring now and then until the cheese has browned, then set aside

4. Spread the almonds on to a baking tray and roast for 6-10 mins. Once done, set aside

5. In a mixing bowl, combine the dressing Ingredients

6. Add the watercress to a salad bowl, top with the roasted pumpkin, halloumi, almonds, avo, drizzle with the salad dressing and serve

Serves: 6

kCal: 456.87 | Carbs: 9.43g | Fat: 25.07g | Protein: 46.33g

INGREDIENTS

- 6oz / 170gr field greens
- 1lb / 454gr feta cheese, chopped
- 2 tablespoons / 28gr butter
- 1 teaspoon / 5gr minced garlic
- 2lb / shrimp
- ½ medium onion, chopped
- 2 medium red peppers, sliced
- 3 teaspoons / 15ml olive oil
- 5 teaspoons / 25ml sugar-free maple syrup
- 2 teaspoons / 10ml apple cider vinegar
- 1 tablespoon / 15ml lemon juice

DIRECTIONS

1. Melt the butter in a pan
2. Add the garlic to the melted butter
3. Add the shrimp and sauté until lightly brown
4. Take off the heat and allow to cool
5. In a salad bowl, mix the field greens, shrimp, feta, onion, and peppers
6. In a mixing bowl, whisk the olive oil, maple syrup, vinegar, and lemon juice
7. Pour the salad dressing onto the salad, and toss until evenly coated

Serves: 6

kCal: 540.38 | Carbs: 3.67g | Fat: 41.9g | Protein: 37.95g

INGREDIENTS

- 6 medium garlic cloves
- 4½ tablespoons / 64gr salted butter
- 4 tablespoons / 60ml Worcestershire sauce
- 2lb / 907gr boneless rib eye
- ½ tablespoon / 4.8gr garlic powder
- 1 tablespoon / 12.19gr ghee
- Salt
- Pepper

DIRECTIONS

1. Preheat a cast iron pan and a separate pan on the stove. Don't add anything to the cast iron pan yet!
2. Mince the garlic and divide intotwo halves
3. Slice the rib eye into strips
4. Add one half of the garlic, garlic powder, salt, and pepper to a mixing bowl and combine
5. Add the rib eye to the garlic mix and coat evenly. Allow to stand for 5 mins
6. Add the ghee to the rib eye and toss to coat
7. In the second pan, fry the second lot of garlic until brown and crisp
8. Add the rib eye to the dry (must be hot and dry) cast iron pan and sear, turning to brown all over
9. Once all seared, add the Worcestershire sauce and butter
10. Allow the butter to melt and then toss to coat the strips evenly
11. Top with the fried garlic

Serves: 6

kCal: 343.33 | Carbs: 4.43g | Fat: 28.7g | Protein: 16.89g

INGREDIENTS

- ¼ cup / 60ml olive oil
- 1 teaspoon / 3.2gr minced garlic
- 1 medium cauliflower, chopped
- 2 cups / 450ml chicken broth
- 1 cup / 237ml water
- 1 cup / 237ml heavy cream
- 1 teaspoon / 5gr xanthan gum
- 1 ½ cups / 350gr grated cheddar
- 4 tablespoons / 28gr bacon bits

DIRECTIONS

1. In a deep pan, ideal for soups, heat up ¾ of the olive oil and garlic on a medium heat
2. Once it's hot, add the chopped cauliflower
3. Up the temp to high, add the broth and water and bring to a boil, stirring frequently
4. As soon as it's boiling add the cream and reduce the temp to medium
5. In a mixing bowl, whisk the rest of the oil and the xanthan gum
6. Drop this mixture into the soup and stir as it thickens
7. Bit by bit, add the cheese, while constantly stirring the soup, so the cheese melts evenly
8. Add the bacon, stir well and serve hot

Serves: 6

kCal: 183.17 | Carbs: 2.41g | Fat: 15.62g | Protein: 6.71g

INGREDIENTS

- 3.53oz / 100gr romaine lettuce
- 2.47oz / 70gr baby spinach
- 1.76oz / 50gr kale
- 6 slices of cooked bacon
- 12 grape tomatoes

- 1 medium avocado, sliced
- 2.12 / 60gr blue cheese
- 3 tablespoons / 36gr sour cream
- 2 ½ tablespoons / 37.5gr mayonnaise

DIRECTIONS

1. In a small bowl, mix the sour cream andmayo together
2. Take half of the cheese and stir into the mayo mixture
3. In a salad bowl, mix all the remaining Ingredients together
4. Divide the salad mixture between serving bowls and top with the mayo / cheese dressing

Serves: 2

kCal: 373.5 | Carbs: 2.83g | Fat: 30.87g | Protein: 19.63g

INGREDIENTS

- 2 Boston lettuce leaves
- ¼oz / 0.62gr fresh basil, finely chopped
- ½ teaspoon / 2.5gr garlic powder
- 1 teaspoon / 5ml lemon juice
- 4 tablespoons / 57.5gr mayonnaise
- 5oz can / 142gr pink salmon, drained
- 1oz / 6.5gr red onion, sliced
- ½ medium avocado, cubed
- 2 tablespoons / 30gr Parmesan cheese, shaved

DIRECTIONS

1. Clean your lettuce leaves well
2. For the spread, combine lemon juice, basil, and garlic powder. Stir well
3. Add the mayo to the spread mixture and set aside to let the flavors grow
4. Fill the lettuce cups with half of the salmon each
5. Add the avo and onion slices on top of the salmon
6. Top each lettuce cup with the spread, and the Parmesan cheese
7. Alternatively, you can use the spread as a dip

Serves: 2

kCal: 891.5 | Carbs: 10.59g | Fat: 61.79g | Protein: 70.68g

INGREDIENTS

- Prep
- 2 chicken breasts
- 2 tablespoons / 30ml olive oil
- Salt
- Pepper
- 10 cherry tomatoes
- 2 medium zucchinis
- Fresh basil for garnishing

- Pesto
- 1 cup / 20gr basil
- ¼ cup / 28.7gr walnuts
- 1 garlic clove
- ½ lemon, zest and juice
- ¼ cup / 22.5gr grated Parmesan
- ¼ cup / 59ml olive oil
- ½ teaspoon / 2.5gr salt

DIRECTIONS

1. Preheat your oven to 400°F / 205°C

2. Place the chicken on a baking sheet, brush with ½ tablespoon of olive oil, season with salt and pepper, and bake for 15 mins

3. Take the chicken out once done, add the tomatoes and brush again with ½ tablespoon olive oil, bake for a further 15 mins until the chicken is cooked through

4. For the pesto, blend together all the Ingredients EXCEPT the olive oil. Once a paste has formed, slowly add the oil while the blender is running on slow. Stop once everything is well combined

5. Spiralize your zucchinis to make the pasta, or use a peeler to make ribbons

6. Add 1 tablespoon of olive oil to a skillet and sauté the zucchini pasta until soft

7. Add the pasta to the pesto

8. Add the pasta to serving bowls, top with the chicken, tomatoes and basil garnish

Serves: 6

kCal: 108.5 | Carbs: 2.82g | Fat: 8.25g | Protein: 5.76g

INGREDIENTS

- 3 large Mexican squash (similar to zucchini)
- 1 teaspoon / 5gr salt
- 3 whole baby Portobello mushrooms, diced
- 1 teaspoon / 5ml olive oil
- 2 teaspoons / 10gr smoked paprika

- 1 tablespoon / 15ml Worcestershire sauce (one without anchovies, check label)
- ½ teaspoon / 2.5gr salt
- 2oz / 55gr grated pepper jack cheese
- 2oz / 55gr grated cheddar
- 3 tablespoons / 23gr sour cream
- 2 tablespoons / 0.9gr chopped chives

DIRECTIONS

1. Preheat your oven to 375°F / 190°C
2. Prepare the squash by removing the ends and slicing lengthways in half
3. With a spoon, carefully scrape out the seeds from each half
4. Sprinkle the skins with salt and allow to sit while drawing excess water. Pat dry
5. In a mixing bowl, add the mushrooms, paprika, ½ tsp salt, Worcestershire sauce and drizzle with oil. Toss to coat evenly
6. Arrange the zucchini and mushrooms on a baking sheet and roast for 8 – 10 mins, until the mushrooms begin to brown
7. Remove from the oven and put the mushrooms into the zucchini skins
8. Top the mushrooms with all the cheeses
9. Bake again for 5 – 10 mins until the cheese melts
10. Top with sour cream and chives

Serves: 4

kCal: 536 | Carbs: 5.82g | Fat: 45.35g | Protein: 24.38g

INGREDIENTS

- 2 medium zucchini
- 1lb / 454gr ground sausage
- 1 cup / 83gr grated cheddar
- ½ medium onion, chopped
- 1 tablespoon / 3gr minced garlic
- 1 teaspoon / 2.5gr paprika
- ½ teaspoon / 1.2gr red pepper flakes
- 1 teaspoon / 1gr dried oregano
- ½ cup / 120ml chicken broth
- Salt
- Pepper

DIRECTIONS

1. Preheat your oven at 350°F / 180°C
2. Slice the zucchinis in half, lengthwise
3. Scoop out the innards to form a "boat"
4. Chop up the zucchini innards
5. Sauté the onions, garlic, and zucchini innards on a medium heat
6. Add in your spices and mix well
7. Turn up the heat to medium-high and add the sausage
8. When the sausage is cooked, add in the cheese and cook until it melts
9. Apportion the sausage mixture equally between the zucchini boats
10. Top with somemore cheese and place in a casserole dish
11. Pour the chicken broth into the bottom of the dish
12. Bake for 30 mins

Serves: 4

kCal: 418.86 | Carbs: 5.62g | Fat: 38.68g | Protein: 12.45g

INGREDIENTS

- 1 tablespoon / 15grbutter
- 1 small onion, chopped
- 2 medium garlic cloves, chopped
- Salt
- Pepper
- ½ teaspoon / 2.5gr xanthan gum
- ½ cup / 120ml chicken broth
- 1 cup / 184gr broccoli, chopped
- 1 cup / 240ml heavy cream
- 1½ cup / 180grgrated cheddar

DIRECTIONS

1. Preheat a soup pot on a medium heat
2. Add the butter, onions, garlic, salt, and pepper to the pot.
3. Sauté until the onions are translucent
4. Sprinkle the xanthan gum over the mixture
5. Add the chicken broth and stir well
6. Add the broccoli and coat everything evenly
7. Add the cream, stirring quickly and frequently, ensuring everything is well mixed and it starts the thicken
8. Add the cheese and whisk until it's melted
9. Serve in soup bowls, garnish with some more broccoli and cheese and serve

Serves: 8

kCal: 382.79 | Carbs: 4.33g | Fat: 25.93g | Protein: 31.85g

INGREDIENTS

- 2 slices bacon, chopped
- 2lb / 910gr of chicken breast fillets (boneless; skinless)
- 16oz / 450gr cream cheese
- ½ cup / 120ml water
- 2 tablespoons / 30ml apple cider vinegar
- 1 tablespoon / 0.45gr dried chives
- 1½ teaspoon / 5gr onion powder
- 1½ teaspoon / 5gr garlic powder
- 1 teaspoon / 2.5gr red pepper flakes, crushed
- 1 teaspoon / 2.5gr dried dill
- Salt
- Pepper
- 2oz / 55gr grated cheddar
- 1 medium green onion, sliced

DIRECTIONS

1 Get out your Instant Pot and set it to sauté and allow to warm up

2. Add the bacon and cook until it's crisp. Remove the bacon, set aside and hit cancel on your Instant Pot

3. Add the chicken, cream cheese, water, vinegar, chives, garlic powder, onion powder, red pepper, dill, salt, and pepper to the Instant Pot

4. Manually set your Instant Pot to high pressure for 15 mins. Do a quick release when done

5. Take out the chicken, shred it and return it to the Instant Pot

6. Add in the cheddar and stir

7. Dish up the chicken, sprinkle with the bacon, and green onion and serve

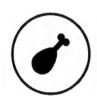

Serves: 6

kCal: 580.17 | Carbs: 3.93g | Fat: 50.74g | Protein: 27.43g

INGREDIENTS

- 6 small strips of bacon
- 2 cups / 470ml heavy whipping cream
- 6oz / 170gr cream cheese
- 1 tablespoon / 14gr butter
- 2 cups / 470ml chicken stock
- 2 cups / 200gr grated Swiss cheese
- 1 cup / 150gr ham, cubed
- 6oz / 170gr shredded chicken breast
- 2 cups / 134gr chopped kale, stems removed

DIRECTIONS

1. Fry the bacon over a medium-low heat until crispy. Roughly chop it and set aside. Reserve about a quarter of the bacon for garnish

2. In a large soup pot, add the cream, butter, cream cheese and cook over a medium heat until everything has melted

3. Add the chicken stock to the soup and simmer

4. Add the grated cheese and stir until it has melted

5. Add the ham, chicken, and ¾ of the bacon to the pot, mix and let simmer

6. Add the kale, stir well and cook for 10 mins until the kale begins to soften

7. Garnish with bacon and serve hot

Serves: 4

kCal: 537.53 | Carbs: 8.21g | Fat: 42.73g | Protein: 31.12g

INGREDIENTS

- 1 small cauliflower, chopped into florets
- 1 cup / 230gr cream cheese
- 1 cup / 230gr grated cheddar
- 4 slices of bacon, chopped
- ¼ cup / 100gr mushrooms, chopped
- 1 medium jalapeno, chopped
- 2 medium chicken thighs, boneless, skinless

DIRECTIONS

1. Preheat your oven to 350°F / 180°C
2. Take out a casserole dish and add the cauli florets
3. To a mixing bowl, add the cream cheese, cheddar, jalapeno, mushrooms, and bacon. Mix well
4. Add the cheese mixture to the cauli florets and mix well
5. Lay out the chicken over the cauli mixture and mix gently
6. Bake for one hour, until the cheese has melted and the chicken is cooked through

Serves: 4

kCal: 562.9 | Carbs: 2.88g | Fat: 40.9g | Protein: 47.75g

INGREDIENTS

- Chicken thighs
- 1½ lb / 680gr chicken thighs, boneless, skinless
- Salt
- Pepper
- 1 tablespoon / 15gr coconut oil
- 4oz / 113gr goats cheese
- 2 tablespoons / 5gr fresh parsley, chopped
- Pepper Sauce
- 4oz / 113gr roasted red peppers
- 2 cloves of garlic
- 2 tablespoons / 30ml olive oil
- ½ cup / 120ml heavy cream

DIRECTIONS

1. Preheat your oven to 350°F / 180°C, and put a skillet on a medium-high heat
2. Season the chicken with the salt and pepper
3. Melt the coconut oil in the skillet and then add the chicken and sear for 5 mins on each side
4. In a blender, add the red peppers, garlic, and olive oil and puree. Add the cream and blend until combined
5. Remove the skillet from the heat, and pour the sauce over the chicken and coat evenly
6. Sprinkle the goats cheese over the chicken
7. Put the skillet in the oven and bake for 10-15mins
8. Garnish with some parsley and serve

Serves: 4

kCal: 315 | Carbs: 2g | Fat: 14g | Protein:42g

INGREDIENTS

- ♦ 2 chicken breasts
- ♦ 1 tablespoon / butter
- ♦ 1 medium onion, diced
- ♦ 1 tablespoon / white wine vinegar
- ♦ 3oz / Gruyere cheese, grated finely
- ♦ 2 tablespoons / fresh sage, finely chopped
- ♦ 1 teaspoon / fresh sage, finely chopped (will make sense in Directions)
- ♦ Salt
- ♦ Pepper

DIRECTIONS

1. Preheat your oven to 375°F / 190°C

2. Line an 11x13" baking pan with parchment paper

3. Butterfly each chicken breast (cutit like you would slice a bagel but not all the way through)

4. With a meat tenderizer, pound the chicken breasts until they are about ¼ inch thick

5. Sprinkle both sides of the chicken breasts with salt and pepper

6. Heat a skillet over a medium heat and add butter

7. Once the butter stops foaming, add the onions and, stirring often, cook until they caramelize

8. Add the vinegar and scrape up the browned bits on the bottom

9. When the vinegar becomes almost syrupy, take the pan off the heat

10. Add the 2 tablespoons of sage and stir well to combine

11. Add the salt and pepper

12. Lay out three pieces of twine and place the chicken breasts on top

13. Spread half the filling on each chicken piece, keeping it away from the edges

14. Sprinkle 2oz of the cheese over the top (keep the last 1oz for later)

15. Roll each breast, being careful not to lose any filling, and secure with the twine (or toothpicks)

16. Place each chicken roll in the baking pan, do not let them touch, and sprinkle the remaining cheese and sage over each one

17. Bake for 35 minutes until the chicken is cooked through. If the chicken isn't properly browned, grill for a few more minutes, but watch carefully as it can burn easily

18. Take out the oven, allow to cool for 5 mins and slice in a crosswise manner, removing the twine

19. Serve warm.

Serves: 4

kCal: 405.25 | Carbs: 4.35g | Fat: 33.94g | Protein: 18.8g

INGREDIENTS

Waffles

- 1½ oz / 44gr cheddar, grated
- 2 large eggs
- 1 cup / 125gr cauliflower crumbles
- ¼ teaspoon / 85gr garlic powder
- ¼ teaspoon / 85gr onion powder

- 4 tablespoons / 24gr almond flour
- 3 tablespoons/ 17gr grated Parmesan
- Salt
- Pepper

Topping

- 4oz / 113gr ground beef
- 4 slices of bacon
- 4 tablespoons / 74gr sugar-free BBQ sauce

- 1½ oz / 44gr cheddar, grated
- Salt
- Pepper

DIRECTIONS

1. Put the cauliflower crumbles into a bowl and add the waffles section of cheddar, parmesan, eggs, almond flour, and spices and set aside

2. Slice the bacon into thin strips and pan fry over a medium-high heat

3. Once the bacon is almost ready, add the beef and cook until crispy

4. Add any excess grease from the pan to the waffle batter

5. Blend your waffle batter into a thick paste.

6. Add half of the waffle mixture to your waffle iron and cook until crisp. Repeat

7. While the waffles are on the go, add the bbq sauce to the bacon and beef in the pan

8. Assemble the waffles together by adding half of the remaining cheese and half of the beef mixture on top of each waffle

9. Grill for 1-2 mins until the cheese has melted and serve hot

Serves: 5

kCal: 493 | Carbs: 5.8g | Fat: 41.2g | Protein: 26g

INGREDIENTS

- 1½ lb / 680gr chicken thighs, bone in, skin on
- 1 lb / 450gr chicken thighs, boneless, skinless
- 2 tablespoons / 30ml olive oil
- 2 teaspoons / 4gr onion powder
- 3 garlic cloves, minced
- 1 inch grated ginger root
- 3 tablespoons / 42gr tomato paste
- 5 teaspoons / 31.5gr Garam Masala
- 2 teaspoons / 4.6gr smoked paprika
- 4 teaspoons / 24gr kosher salt
- 10oz can / 284gr can diced tomatoes
- 1 cup / 237ml heavy cream
- 1 cup / 237ml coconut milk
- 1 teaspoon / 3.3gr Guar gum
- Fresh cilantro for garnish

DIRECTIONS

1. De-bone the boned chicken thighs and chop all the chicken into bite-sized pieces
2. Add the chicken to the slow cooker and grate the ginger over the top
3. Add all the dry spices
4. Add the can of tomatoes, olive oil, tomato paste and mix well
5. Add ½ of the coconut milk and mix thoroughly
6. Cook on low for 6 hours or on high for 3 hours
7. Once done, add the remaining coconut milk, cream, guar gum and mix well into the chicken
8. Serve with your choice of sides

Serves: 2

kCal: 325.5 | Carbs: 11.46g | Fat: 26.08g | Protein: 10.65g

INGREDIENTS

Zucchini Pasta

- 3 medium zucchini
- ½ teaspoon / 3gr salt
- Avo-Walnut Pesto
- ½ large avocado
- 1 cup / 20gr fresh basil leaves
- ¼ cup / 29gr walnuts
- 2 garlic cloves, peeled
- ½ large lemon
- ¼ cup / 22.5gr grated Parmesan
- ½ cup / 118ml water, if needed

Other

- 1 tablespoon / 15ml olive oil
- 5-6 fresh basil leaves for garnish
- Salt
- Pepper

DIRECTIONS

1. Preheat Cut the zucchini into ribbons with a peeler. Stop peeling once you reach the seeds
2. Place the ribbons in a colander and toss with the salt. Allow to stand
3. Add all the pesto Ingredients to a food processor and blend until smooth
4. Add the water to thin the pesto, if required
5. Grease a skillet with olive oil and bring to a medium heat
6. Sauté the zucchini ribbons for 3 – 5 mins and remove from the heat
7. Spoon the pesto overthe zucchini and gently toss to coat
8. Divide equally between two plates and garnish with fresh basil and Parmesan

Serves: 5

kCal: 295.4 | Carbs: 5.35g | Fat: 18.66g | Protein: 28.26g

INGREDIENTS

Meatballs

- ♦ 1lb / 454gr ground beef
- ♦ 1 large egg
- ♦ ¼ cup / 59gr Parmesan cheese
- ♦ ½ teaspoon / 1gr onion powder

Sauce

- ♦ 1½ cups / 355ml water
- ♦ ¼ cup / 58gr apple cider vinegar
- ♦ 3 tablespoons / 45ml soy sauce
- ♦ ⅓ cup / 78gr sugar-free ketchup
- ♦ 1 cup / 200gr erythritol
- ♦ ½ teaspoon / 2.5gr xanthan gum

DIRECTIONS

1. In a large mixing bowl, add all the meatball Ingredients and combine well with your hands

2. Use a tablespoon to measure and shape your meatballs. You should end up with around 30 mini meatballs

3. Preheat a saucepan on a medium heat and cook the meatballs until browned on the outside. Put aside

4. In the same saucepan, add everything for the sauce, except the xanthan gum and whisk together well

5. Slowly whisk in the xanthan gum, a little at a time

6. Lower the temperature and simmer on low

7. After a few minutes, check if you're happy with the consistency. Should not slide off the back of a spoon.

8. Add the meatballs to the sauce and simmer on low for 10 minutes.

9. Serve with whatever you desire, eg: cauli rice

Serves: 8

kCal: 509.8 | Carbs:8.5g | Fat: 32.99g | Protein: 41.14g

INGREDIENTS

- ◆ 2 tablespoons / 28.2gr butter
- ◆ 1 medium onion, diced
- ◆ 10 medium chicken thighs, boneless, skinless, cubed
- ◆ 14oz / 397gr canned diced green chilies
- ◆ 2 teaspoons / 12gr salt
- ◆ 2 teaspoons / 4gr cumin
- ◆ 2 teaspoons / 3.6gr oregano
- ◆ 1 teaspoon / black pepper
- ◆ 1lb / 454gr frozen cauliflower
- ◆ 4 cups / 960ml chicken broth
- ◆ 2 cups / 490gr sour cream
- ◆ 1 cup / 237ml heavy whipping cream

DIRECTIONS

1. Turn on your Instant Pot to the sautée setting and melt the butter
2. Add the onion and chicken
3. Cook until the chicken is mostly done
4. Add the chilies, salt, cumin, oregano, pepper and cauliflower and stir well
5. Add the chicken broth
6. Close the Instant Pot and cook on high pressure for 30 mins
7. Let the Instant Pot sit for 10 mins before releasing the steam and opening it
8. Whisk in the creams and serve immediately

Serves: 6

kCal: 338 | Carbs: 2.56g | Fat: 18.28g | Protein: 37.96g

INGREDIENTS

- 4oz / 113gr cream cheese
- ⅓ cup / 75gr grated mozzarella
- 10oz / 284gr package of frozen spinach, thawed
- 3 whole chicken breasts
- 1 tablespoon / 15ml olive oil

- ⅔ cup / 150gr tomato basil sauce (preferably Rao's)
- 3oz / 85gr mozzarella slices
- Salt
- Pepper

DIRECTIONS

1. Preheat your oven to 400°F / 204°C

2. In a microwave-safe bowl, add the cream cheese, mozzarella, and spinach and heat for about 2 mins, until the cheeses start to melt. Mix it all in and add salt and pepper

3. Cut several slices across each chicken breast, cutting as deeply as you can without cutting all the way through

4. Season the chicken with salt and pepper

5. Stuff each chicken breast with the cheese mixture

6. Brush some olive oil over the tops of the chicken and cook in the oven for 25 minutes, or until the chicken reaches 165°F/ 74°C

7. Change your oven to grill, add the basil sauce and mozzarella slices to the chicken

8. Grill for 5 mins, until the cheese starts to melt and brown

Serves: 8

kCal: 230.28 | Carbs: 3.85g | Fat: 17.6g | Protein: 12.52g

INGREDIENTS

Rolls

- 8 large cabbage leaves
- 8oz / 227gr pastrami, chopped
- 1 ½ cups / 162gr grated Swiss cheese
- ½ cup / 71gr drained sauerkraut
- Thousand Island Dressing
- ½ cup / 14gr mayonnaise
- ¼ cup / 59gr sugar-free ketchup
- 1 garlic clove, minced
- 2 tablespoons / 37gr Sriracha sauce
- 1 teaspoon / 2.3gr onion powder
- Salt
- Pepper

DIRECTIONS

1. Preheat your oven to 350°F / 180°C, and boil some water
2. Place the cabbage into a large bowl and pour the boiling water over them. Leave them for 3-5 mins, take them out of the water and set aside
3. In a mixing bowl, add the mayo, ketchup, garlic, lemon juice, sriracha, onion powder, salt, and pepper and mix well to make the dressing
4. In another bowl, mix together the pastrami, cheese, sauerkraut, and half of the dressing
5. Lay one cabbage leaf out and spoon 1/8 of the meat mixture in the center. Roll it up like you would a burrito. Place the roll seam side down into a baking dish. Repeat with all the leaves
6. Spread the rest of the dressing over the cabbage burritos and then bake for 30 mins

Serves: 4

kCal: 375.75 | Carbs: 8.37g | Fat: 28.07g | Protein: 19.27g

INGREDIENTS

- 1 large eggplant, sliced into 8 ½ inch slices
- Lots of Salt (keep the salt pot with you)
- 1 large egg
- ½ cup / 45gr grated Parmesan
- ¼ cup / 55gr ground pork rinds
- ½ tablespoon / 3.2gr Italian seasoning
- 1 cup / 270gr tomato sauce
- ½ cup / 113gr grated mozzarella
- 4 tablespoons / 60ml melted butter

DIRECTIONS

1. Preheat your oven to 400°F / 205°C
2. Line a baking sheet with a paper towel and place the eggplant slices on top. Sprinkle both sides of each slice with salt. Leave it for 30 mins while the excess moisture is released
3. Combine the pork rinds, parmesan, and Italian seasoning in a bowl and set aside
4. Beat the egg and place next to the pork rinds so you can work quickly
5. Pour the melted butter into a 9x13 inch baking dish
6. Pat the eggplant dry and dip each slice into the egg and then into the pork rind mixture, covering entirely with crumbs.
7. Place each crumbed slice into the melted butter
8. Bake for 20 mins. Flip each slice over and bake for a further 20 mins, until golden brown
9. Top the eggplant with the tomato sauce and the mozzarella
10. Bake for a further 5 mins until the cheese has melted

Serves: 5

kCal: 110.96 | Carbs: 3.88g | Fat: 4.43g | Protein: 10.43g

INGREDIENTS

Ramen

- 1 tablespoon/ 15ml olive oil
- 1 small onion, thinly sliced
- 1 tablespoon / 6gr freshly grated ginger
- 3 garlic cloves, finely minced
- 1 teaspoon / 5gr chili paste
- 1 tablespoon / 15ml fish sauce
- ¼ cup / 60ml soy sauce
- ¼ cup / 60ml rice wine vinegar
- 4oz / 113gr mushrooms, thinly sliced
- Salt
- Pepper
- 5 cups / 1.2L beef broth
- 3 packets of shiritaki noodles
- 10 slices of roast beef

Optional toppings

- Hard-boiled eggs
- Cilantro
- Sesame seeds
- Chopped green onion
- Extra chili sauce
- Seaweed flakes

DIRECTIONS

1. Heat the oil in a large soup pot, overa medium heat.
2. Add the onions and cook until soft
3. Add the ginger, garlic, chili paste, fish sauce, soy sauce, vinegar, mushrooms, salt, pepper, and beef broth and simmer for 30 mins
4. Rinse the noodles under cold water and add to the pot
5. Taste test and add salt if needed
6. Divide the noodles and broth into serving bowls
7. Add the beef and then the optional toppings as desired

Serves: 24

kCal: 72.71 | Carbs: 1.67g | Fat: 6.97g | Protein: 1.23g

INGREDIENTS

- 16oz / 450gr softened cream cheese
- 2 cup / 60gr unsweetened cocoa powder, divided in half
- 4 tablespoons / 50gr erythritol
- ¼ teaspoon / 1.2ml liquid stevia
- ½ teaspoon / 2.5ml rum extract
- 1 tablespoon / 3.5gr instant coffee
- 2 tablespoons / 30ml water
- 1 tablespoon / 15ml heavy whipping cream
- 24 paper candy cups

DIRECTIONS

1. Add to a large mixing bowl everything except one half of the cocoa powder

2. With a hand mixer, whip everything together until well combined and put in the fridge for 30 mins to chill

3. Sprinkle out the remaining cocoa powder

4. Take a tablespoon of the chilled mixture and, using your hands, roll into a ball, then roll int the cocoa powder

5. Repeat until you have used all the mixture. You should end up with around 24 balls

6. Place each ball in a paper cup

7. Keep in the fridge until ready to serve

Serves: 2

kCal: 349.35 | Carbs: 5.75g | Fat: 33.15g | Protein: 7.2g

INGREDIENTS

- 1oz / 28gr 70% dark chocolate
- 2 tablespoons / 20gr hulled hemp seeds
- 2 tablespoons / 15gr powdered erythritol
- 1 tablespoon / 6.25gr cacao powder
- ½ cup / 120ml coconut cream, chilled
- ½ medium avocado
- ½ cup / 120ml almond milk
- 1 cup ice

DIRECTIONS

1 Add the chocolate, cacao, erythritol, and hemp seeds to a blender and pulse blend to chop up the chocolate

2. Add all the rest of the Ingredients and blend until smooth and then serve

Serves: 1

kCal: 369 | Carbs: 7.53g | Fat: 34.95g | Protein: 8.1g

INGREDIENTS

- 1 cup / 240ml coconut milk
- 7 ice cubes
- 2 tablespoons / 30gr peanut butter
- 2 tablespoons / 30ml sugar-free salted caramel syrup
- 1 tablespoon / 15ml MCT oil
- ¼ teaspoon / 2.5gr xanthan gum

DIRECTIONS

1 Add everything to a blender and blend until the consistency is perfect for you

2. Serve as desired and feel free to sprinkle cocoa powder for garnish

Serves: 1

kCal: 346 | Carbs: 4.8g | Fat: 34.17g | Protein: 2.62g

INGREDIENTS

- 7 ice cubes
- 1 cup/ 240ml unsweetened coconut milk
- ¼ cup / 36gr blackberries
- 2 tablespoons / 15gr cocoa powder
- 12 drops of liquid stevia
- ¼ teaspoon / 1.2gr xanthan gum
- 2 tablespoons / 30ml MCT oil

DIRECTIONS

I   Add everything to a blender and blend until everything is well combined

Serves: 25

kCal: 145.32 | Carbs: 1.83g | Fat: 12.96g | Protein: 3.58g

INGREDIENTS

- Chocolate layer
- 1 ¼ cups / 300ml heavy whipping cream
- ½ cup / 62.5gr powdered erythritol
- ½ teaspoon / 2.5ml liquid stevia
- ½ teaspoon / 2.5ml vanilla extract
- 6oz / 120gr unsweetened chocolate, chopped
- PB layer
- 1 cup / 240gr creamy peanut butter
- ¼ cup / 31.2gr powdered erythritol
- ½ teaspoon / 2.5ml vanilla extract

DIRECTIONS

1 Line a baking dish with baking paper

2. Grease the baking paper too, to make it easier to remove later

3. Preheat a saucepan on a medium heat and add these chocolate layer Ingredients: sweeteners, vanilla, and cream

4. Bring to a simmer and take off the heat. Add the chocolate and allow to soften for 5 mins

5. Whisk to dissolve the chocolate

6. Pour half of the chocolate mixture into the prepared baking dish, making sure it's evenly spread to the edges and chill in the freezer for 20 mins

7. Keep the other half of the chocolate mixture warm while the rest is chilling

8. Heat the peanut butter in the microwave in 30 sec spurts until it's melted

9. Add the sweetener and vanilla to the peanut butter

10. Pour the peanut butter over the chilled chocolate layer and freeze until firm

11. Add the remaining chocolate as the top layer and put in the fridge until set.

12. Cut into small squares and serve

Serves: 12

kCal: 217.14 | Carbs: 3.56g | Fat: 19.47g | Protein: 7.65g

INGREDIENTS

Cream Cheese Filling
- 6oz / 162gr softened cream cheese
- 3 tablespoons / 23gr powdered erythritol
- 1 tablespoon / 15ml heavy cream
- ½ teaspoon / 2.5ml vanilla extract

Muffins
- 2 cups / 192gr almond flour
- ½ cup / 100gr erythritol
- ¼ cup / 50gr unflavored whey protein powder
- 2 teaspoons / 10gr baking powder
- 2 teaspoons / 4gr pumpkin pie spice
- ½ teaspoon / 2.5gr salt
- 2 large eggs
- ½ cup / 123gr pumpkin puree
- ¼ cup / 56gr melted butter
- ¼ cup / 60ml unsweetened almond milk
- ½ teaspoon / 2.5gr vanilla extract

DIRECTIONS

1. Preheat your oven to 325°F/ 160°C
2. Mix all the cream cheese filling Ingredients until you get a smooth batter
3. In another mixing bowl, whisk the almond flour, sweetener, protein powder, baking powder, spice and salt
4. Add the eggs, pumpkin puree, butter, milk, and vanilla and mix well
5. Grease a muffin pan and add a spoonful of batter to each muffin well
6. Use a spoon to make a hole in the middle and add cream cheese filling to each hole
7. Top each muffin with muffin batter
8. Bake for 25 mins until the muffins are cooked in the middle (use the toothpick method)
9. Allow to cool beforetaking them out of the muffin pan

Serves: 64

kCal: 121.94 | Carbs: 1.92g | Fat: 11.85g | Protein: 2.32g

INGREDIENTS

- 1½ cups / 144gr almond flour
- 2½ cups / 312gr powdered erythritol
- 5 tablespoons / 71gr butter, melted
- 1lb / 454gr softened cream cheese

- 15 whole mint leaves
- ¼ cup / 60ml heavy cream
- 6oz / 70% dark chocolate
- ¼ teaspoon / 1.2ml mint extract

DIRECTIONS

1. Preheat your oven to 350°F / 180°C
2. Line a square baking tin with baking paper
3. In a large mixing bowl add the flour and half a cup of the sweetener and mix well
4. Add the melted butter to the bowl, and mix until a dough forms
5. Press the dough into the baking tin and bake until light brown (about 8 mins)
6. Remove from the pan and allow to cool
7. In a mixer, beat the cream cheese and remaining sweetener. Once done, set aside
8. Add the mint and the cream to a blender and blend until smooth
9. Add the mint cream mix to the cream cheese filling and fold together
10. Spread the mint and cream cheese mix over the cooled crust
11. Put in the freezer for about 3 hours until firm
12. Oncefirm, cut into 64 pieces and return to the freezer
13. Melt the chocolate until thin and add the mint extract
14. Top each square with the chocolate, however you like, and allow to cool

Serves: 10

kCal: 55.4 | Carbs: 0g | Fat: 0g | Protein: 0.8g

INGREDIENTS

- 1 cup / 240ml water
- 5 teaspoons (2 envelopes) / 23gr unflavored gelatine
- ½ teaspoon coconut extract
- ⅓ cup / 65gr powdered erythritol
- 1 cup 80% proof rum (or a low carb alcohol alternative you might prefer)
- 2oz Containers with lids for easy stacking and storing
- Optional toppings: whipped cream, raspberries

DIRECTIONS

1. Heat up half of the water until quite hot and add the gelatine
2. Stir in the rest of the water and allow to cool, but don't let it cool too much as it will start to firm
3. Add the coconut extract and erythritol and mix well
4. Do a taste test and add more erythritol if needed
5. Stir in the rum (or your preferred alternative)
6. Pour the jello mix into the containers and place in the fridge to set
7. Serve plain or with toppings of your choice

Having a meal plan for even the week ahead can eliminate a lot of temptations for you. Often we rush home from work or school and we have to make dinner in a rush, so we grab the quick things like pasta, or the ever easy takeout option.

If you just take some of your rare free moments and plan ahead, you can get your choice meals ready before hand and you will feel all the better for it. And so will your scale!

Herewith is a 14-Day meal plan, consisting of recipes from this book, and one new one per day. You don't have to stick to it 100% either. Mix and match to whatever you prefer, just make a plan to stick to it, especially if you're committed to losing weight. The next step after you've decided on your meal plan, is to go through your groceries. Go through each recipe and see what you have and what you still need, make a grocery list, and then hit the grocery store. Keto does involve a lot of dedication and cooking on your part. If you know your week is busy, do some of the baking on the weekend, so you can just pack up your lunch and go. Or pop the prepped dinner in the oven to be ready in 30mins instead of an hour. If one or two meals requires a bit of veggie prep, prepare the veg at a time when you can and store it in the fridge for when you're ready.

If you're serious about doing keto, you can make it work. All the recipes are super easy to do, so find the ones that fit in with your lifestyle and watch the pounds drop!

*indicates a new meal not mentioned in this book

DAY 1

Breakfast*: Blueberry Ricotta Pancakes

Serves 5 | kCal: 311.4 | Carbs: 5.78g | Fat: 22.61g | Prot: 15.25g

INGREDIENTS

- 3 large eggs
- ¾ cup / 200gr ricotta
- ½ teaspoon / 2.5gr vanilla extract
- ¼ cup / 60ml unsweetened vanilla almond milk
- 1 cup / 130gr almond flour
- ½ cup / 65gr golden flaxseed meal
- ¼ teaspoon / 2gr salt
- 1 teaspoon / 5gr baking powder
- ¼ teaspoon / 2gr stevia
- ¼ cup / 85gr blueberries

DIRECTIONS

1. Put a skillet on a medium heat
2. Blend together the eggs, ricotta, vanilla extract and milk
3. In another mixing bowl, add the flour, flaxseed, salt, baking powder, and stevia and combine
4. Carefully add the dry Ingredients to the wet and blend until smooth
5. Melt the butter in the pan
6. Scoop the batter in 2 tbsp measures and pour into thepan
7. Add 3 to 4 blueberries to each pancake
8. Once lightly browned, flip and cook the other side
9. Serve with whatever low carb topping you wish

Lunch: Avo Bowls (See page 41)

Dinner: Eggplant Parmesan (See page 70)

MEAL PREP TIPS & TRICKS

1. For breakfast, make your batter the night before, so all you need to do in the morning, is cook

2. For lunch, and dinner, prep everything during some down time

DAY 2

Breakfast: Pizza eggs (See page 25)

Lunch*: Cheezy Peppers

Serves 4 | kCal: 245.5 | Carbs:5.97g| Fat:16.28g | Prot:17.84g

INGREDIENTS

- 4 large eggs
- 2 medium bell peppers
- ½ cup / 170gr ricotta
- ½ cup / 170gr grated mozzarella
- ½ cup / 170gr grated parmesan
- 1 teaspoon / 5gr garlic powder
- ¼ teaspoon / 2gr dried parsley
- ¼ cup / 85gr baby spinach leaves
- 2 tablespoons / 28grextra parmesan for garnish

DIRECTIONS

1. Preheat oven to 375°F / 190°C
2. Slice the peppers in half and remove seeds
3. Add the cheeses, eggs, garlic powder and parsley to a blender and mix well
4. Pour the mixture into each pepper half
5. Add spinach leaves and push them into thestuffing
6. Line a baking sheet and place the peppers
7. Cover with foil and bake for 35 – 45 mins
8. Sprinkle with remaining parmesan and grill until the tops brown

Dinner: Cheesy Broccoli Soup (See page 56)

MEAL PREP TIPS & TRICKS

1. If you really enjoy the Pizza Eggs, make extra to take for lunch, saving you some time.
2. Swapping meals around is perfectly acceptable!

DAY 3

Breakfast: Coconut Berry Porridge (See page 22)

Lunch: Bacon & Blue Cheese Salad (See page 50)

Dinner*: Philly Cheesesteak

Serves 5 | kCal: 535.74 | Carbs: 8.72g | Fat: 35.64g | Prot: 42.74g

INGREDIENTS

- 1 tablespoon / 15ml olive oil
- 1 medium onion, cut in half
- 2 teaspoons / 10gr minced garlic
- 1 cup / 250gr green bell pepper, diced
- 1lb / 455gr ground beef
- 1 teaspoon / 5gr salt
- ¼ teaspoon / 2gr black pepper
- ¼ teaspoon / 2grgarlic powder
- ¼ teaspoon / 2gr onion powder
- ¼ cup / 120ml beef broth
- 1lb / 455gr cauliflower florets
- 8oz / 227gr sliced mushrooms
- ¼ cup/ 120ml half and half
- 10 slices provolone cheese

DIRECTIONS

1. Dice one half of the onion and thinly slice the other
2. Add the olive oil to a large skillet. Once heated, add the onion slices, garlic, and half bell pepper
3. Sauté until the veggies soften
4. Add the beef, onion powder, garlic powder, salt, and half of the black pepper
5. Crumble the beef with amasher
6. Cover the skillet and cook for a few more minutes, stirring occasionally until the beef is cooked
7. Add the beef broth, cauliflower, onions, peppers, mushrooms, and stir
8. Allow to simmer for 15 minutes and then mash the cauliflower
9. Turn off the heat and add the half and half. Stir to mix well

10. Season with the remaining seasonings

11. Lay the cheese slices over the top and cover with a lid

12. Cook until the cheese melts

MEAL PREP TIPS & TRICKS

I   Philly Cheesesteak is the perfect meal to have as leftovers the next day! More time saved!

DAY 4

Breakfast*: Chorizo Eggs

Serves 4 | kCal: 321 | Carbs: 2.02g | Fat: 27.31g | Prot: 15.57g

INGREDIENTS

- ♦ 5 large eggs
- ♦ 2oz / 56gr chorizo
- ♦ 2 tablespoons / 28grbutter
- ♦ Salt
- ♦ Pepper

- ♦ ⅔ cup / 85gr grated pepper jack cheese
- ♦ 1 medium avocado
- ♦ 2 tablespoons / 28gr sour cream
- ♦ 2 tablespoons / 28grcilantro, chopped *Optional garnish

DIRECTIONS

1. Preheat oven to 400°F/ 205°C
2. Preheat an oven-safe skillet on a medium heat
3. Remove the chorizo meat from the casings and add it to the skillet
4. Fry until cooked and allow to drain on some paper towels
5. Melt the butter in the skillet and ensure the whole pan is evenly coated
6. Take off the heat and place on a heat-proof surface
7. Add the eggs to the buttered pan and sprinkle with salt and pepper
8. Add some of the cooked chorizo on the eggs and sprinkle evenly with cheese
9. Place the pan in the oven for 15 – 20 mins, until the cheese bubbles
10. Serve warm with avo, sour cream, and optional cilantro

Lunch: Pizza Dogs (See page 44)

Dinner: Chicken de la Crème (See page 57)

MEAL PREP TIPS & TRICKS

I Pizza Dogs are best made on slower days, but are the perfect grab-and-go meal

DAY 5

Breakfast: Maple Muffins (See page 33)

Lunch*: Steak Stroganoff

Serves 1 | kCal: 594.52 | Carbs: 6.9g | Fat: 49g | Prot: 33.1g

INGREDIENTS

- 1 tablespoon / 15gr butter
- Salt
- Pepper
- 4oz / 114gr rib eye steak
- 4oz / 114gr whole mushrooms, cut into quarters
- 1 large clove of garlic, minced
- 3 tablespoons / 45ml chicken stock
- 1½oz / 43gr cream cheese
- ¼ teaspoon / 2ml Worcestershire sauce
- ¼ teaspoon / 2gr black pepper
- 1 teaspoon/ 5gr minced parsley

DIRECTIONS

1. Preheat a skillet on a medium-high heat and add half of the butter
2. Add the steak, season with salt and pepper, and sear. Set aside
3. Add the remaining butter to the pan, and once melted, cook the mushrooms until softened
4. Reduce the heat to low, add the garlic and cook for another minute
5. Add the stock, and make sure you scrape all the bits at the bottom
6. Add the cheese, Worcestershire sauce, black pepper and stir until the cheese has melted
7. Plate the steak, pour the sauce over and garnish with the parsley

Dinner: Chicken Marinara (See page 68)

MEAL PREP TIPS & TRICKS

1. These breakfast muffins are the best example for weekend meal prep. As this recipe makes so many, keep them around for those times when you have run out of time. Also a great lunch box filler!

DAY 6

Breakfast: Zucchini Walnut Bread (See page 38)

Lunch: Cauli-Bacon Soup (See page 49)

Dinner*: Chicken Salad

Serves 4 | kCal: 725.12 | Carbs: 5.38g | Fat: 57.29g | Prot: 37.85g

INGREDIENTS

- 2 tablespoons / 24gr olive oil
- 1.1oz / 500gr chicken breasts, cut into cubes
- 1 garlic clove, minced
- 1cup / 65gr mushrooms, sliced
- ⅓ cup / 43gr fresh basil
- 5oz / 140gr fresh spinach
- 3-4 small sun-dried tomatoes
- 1 cup / 235ml sugar-free ranch dressing

DIRECTIONS

1. Add the olive oil in a pan on a medium heat
2. Once hot, add the chicken and cook until brown
3. Just before the chicken is ready, add the garlic and stir well
4. Once the chicken is done, put it in a mixing bowl and set aside
5. Add bacon to the same pan, cook until it's at your preferred crispiness, then add to the chicken
6. Add the mushrooms, basil and some of the spinach to the chicken and mix well
7. Add the remaining spinach to a salad bowl, spread the chicken salad over thetop
8. Garnish with the tomatoes and ranch dressing

MEAL PREP TIPS & TRICKS

1. Soups are an excellent meal to prep over the weekend. Not only that, you can have them for lunch or dinner.

DAY 7

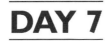

Breakfast*: Breakfast Bowl

Serves 4 | kCal: 887.68 | Carbs: 8.2g | Fat: 75.4g | Prot: 40.95g

INGREDIENTS

- 1lb / 450gr beef sirloin
- ¼ cup / 59ml soy sauce
- 2 tablespoons / 30ml Calamansi juice (Filipino lemonade)
- 6 medium garlic cloves, minced
- 3 teaspoons / 14gr garlic powder
- 1 tablespoon / 14gr erythritol
- 1 cup / 128gr coconut oil
- 1lb / 455gr cauliflower rice
- 4 large eggs
- Salt
- Pepper

DIRECTIONS

1 Combine the soy sauce, Calamansi juice, some of the garlic, some of the garlic powder, erythritol, salt, and pepper together and mix until everything is dissolved

2. Put the meat into a Ziploc bag and pour the marinade over the beef

3. Seal the bag and refrigerate overnight

4. The following day, remove the meat from the bag

5. Coat a frying pan with some of the oil, heat, add the beef and fry until all the liquid is almost gone

6. Keep turning the beef

7. Take the beef off the heat, allow to cool before cutting into strips

8. Add the remaining oil, garlic, garlic powder, and some salt to the pan and sauté until aromatic

9. Add the cauliflower rice and coat well, cooking until tender

10. Fry the eggs as you prefer, in a separate frying pan

11. Layer a bowl with the rice, beef, top with the eggs and serve

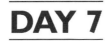

Lunch: Taco Salad (See page 42)

Dinner: Roast Chicken in Pepper Sauce (See page 60)

MEAL PREP TIPS & TRICKS

1 Calamansi juice might not be easily accessible, so feel free to substitute it with a sugar-free version.

2. As with any recipe, feel free to substitute for foods you would prefer, just keep in mind they need to be keto-friendly.

DAY 8

Breakfast: Breakfast Burger (See page 26)

Lunch*: Eggs Benedict Salad

Serves 3 | kCal: 333.63 | Carbs: 2.5g | Fat: 31.73g | Prot: 14.77g

INGREDIENTS

- 3 strips of bacon
- 3 tables poons / 27grgrated parmesan
- 3 cups / 550gr spring mix greens
- 6 cherry tomatoes, halved
- 2 medium egg yolks
- ¼ cup / 55gr butter
- 1 teaspoon / 5ml lemon juice
- 3 medium eggs, poached
- 1 tablespoon / 0.45gr dried chives

DIRECTIONS

1. Fry bacon as desired and allow to cool
2. Spray cooking spray onto a microwave-safe plate
3. On the plate, place the parmesan cheese in 3 heaps and microwave until crispy. Allow to cool
4. In a blender, add egg yolks, and lemon juice and blend until pale yellow
5. Microwave the butter until it starts to bubble. Add to the blender and combine until light in color
6. Plate the greens, tomatoes and bacon, add a layer of parmesan, and then the poached eggs
7. Pour your hollandaise sauce over everything
8. Garnish with chives

Dinner: Zucchini Pasta (See page 65)

MEAL PREP TIP & TRICKS

1 The burger calls for PB Fit powder, but don't panic if you can't find it. You can sub some regular, sugar-free peanut butter instead. This is also quite a heavy breakfast, so if you find yourself not hungry come lunch time, have a slice of Zuccini Bread or a Maple Muffin or two.

2. If you're a pasta lover, it might be a good idea to make a lot of zucchini ribbons and store them for future use.

DAY 9

Breakfast: Bacon and Eggs (See page 29)

Lunch: Casserole Sub Sandwich (See page 40)

Dinner*: Unreal Crab Cakes

Serves 3 | kCal: 434.24 | Carbs: 5.47g | Fat: 41.01g | Prot:10.03g

INGREDIENTS

- 1 can of hearts of palm, liquid drained
- 2 tablespoons / 30ml mayonnaise
- 1 teaspoon / 5gr Old Bay seasoning
- 1 tablespoon / 1gr of parsley
- ¼ cup / 32gralmond flour
- 1 large egg, beaten
- 1 tablespoon / 10gr diced onion
- 1 teaspoon / 5gr butter
- 3 tablespoons / 42gr almond meal
- 2 tablespoons / 18gr parmesan cheese
- 4 tablespoons / 60ml avocado oil

DIRECTIONS

1. With a fork, shred the hearts of palm until it resembles crab meat
2. Add the seasoning, mayo, almond flour, egg, and parsley, and mix until well combined
3. In a skillet, melt the butter on a medium heat and sauté the onion until it's soft
4. Gently fold the onions into the"crab meat"
5. In a bowl, mix the almond meal and parmesan to make a coating mixture
6. Divide the "crab meat" into 6 equal balls and press into the coating mixture
7. Squash the balls to form cakes and ensure they are completely coated
8. Heat a skillet over a medium-high heat and add the avo oil

9. Fry each cake until browned on each side

10. Serve hot

MEAL PREP TIPS & TRICKS

I Don't stress too much about the mayo in some of these recipes. There are sugar-free options, just remember to check the labels.

DAY 10

Breakfast*: Pancake Bites with Blueberries

Serves 6 | kCal: 174.77 | Carbs: 7.07g | Fat: 13.27g | Prot: 6.52g

INGREDIENTS

- 4 large eggs
- ¼ cup / 85gr erythritol
- ½ teaspoon / 2.5ml vanilla extract
- ½ cup / 170gr of coconut flour
- ¼ cup / 85gr butter, melted
- 1 teaspoon / 5gr baking powder
- ½ teaspoon / 2.5gr salt
- ¼ teaspoon / 2gr cinnamon
- ⅓ cup / 80ml water
- ½ cup / 170gr frozen blueberries

DIRECTIONS

1. Preheat the oven to 325°F / 165°C
2. Greaseproof a muffin tin. Make sure it's done well, as the batter is very sticky
3. Mix the eggs, erythritol, and vanilla extract in a blender
4. Add the flour, melted butter, baking powder, salt, and cinnamon and blend until smooth
5. Rest the batter for a bit to thicken up
6. Add the water one-third at a time, blending after each addition
7. Blend until the batter is thick enough to be scooped but not poured
8. Fill each muffin well with the batter, add some blueberries, and push them into the batter
9. Bake for 25 mins. Use the toothpick test to see if they're ready
10. Serve with your choice of low-carb toppings

Lunch: Breaded Chicken Pieces (See page 45)

Dinner: Bacon BBQ Pizza Waffles (See page 63)

MEAL PREP TIPS & TRICKS

| Fill your freezer with loads of frozen berries! There's so many different ways to use them: toppings, smoothies, baking, and more!

DAY 11

Breakfast: Ham Souffle (See page 101)

Lunch*: Pressed Halloumi

Serves 1 | kCal: 434 | Carbs: 5.7g | Fat: 32.3g | Prot: 27.6g

INGREDIENTS

- 4oz / 115gr halloumi
- 2 teaspoons / 9.5gr of mayonnaise
- ¼ cup / 45gr spinach
- 4 leaves of basil, torn
- 0.8oz / 23gr ofcucumber, sliced
- 6 whole blackberries, sliced in half

DIRECTIONS

1. Warm up your Panini press tomedium
2. Slice the halloumi into 2 equal-sized rectangles
3. Cook the halloumi on the press until it starts to brown
4. Flip and repeat on the other side
5. On one halloumi slice, layer the mayo, spinach, cucumber, basil, and blackberries
6. Place the other slice on top of the fillings to make a sandwich
7. Close the pressfor one minute
8. Plate the sandwich and top with and remaining berries
9. Serve warm

Dinner: Cabbage Burritos (See page 69)

MEAL PREP TIPS & TRICKS

1. If you don't have a Panini press, simply use a frying pan and a spatula and just keep flipping until it's perfect.

DAY 12

Breakfast: Pancake Sandwich (See page 27)

Lunch: Pumpkin Halloumi Salad (See page 46)

Dinner*: Instant Pot Lasagne

Serves 8 | kCal: 403.24 | Carbs: 7.36g | Fat: 26.85g | Prot: 30.9g

INGREDIENTS

- 1lb / 450gr ground beef
- 2 garlic cloves, minced
- 1 small onion, diced
- 1½ cup / 340gr ricotta
- ½ cup / 70gr parmesan
- 2 large eggs
- 25oz / 740ml marinara sauce
- 8oz / 230grsliced mozzarella
- 1 cup / 235ml water

DIRECTIONS

1 Set the Instant Pot to the sauté setting and brown the beef, garlic, and onion

2. Mix the ricotta, parmesan, and eggs together well

3. Switch off the Instant Pot, remove the beef and drain the grease

4. Add the marinara to the beef and mix thoroughly. Leave some sauce for topping

5. Wrap the base of a spring-form pan with foil. Make sure the pan can fit into the Instant Pot

6. Layer as follows in the spring-form pan: Meat, mozzarella, ricotta mix, until everything is in

7. Top off with the remaining marinara

8. Cover the pan loosely with some foil

9. Add the water to the Instant Pot, then the rack, and then the spring-form pan onto the rack

10. Close the Instant Pot lid and valve and cook on high pressure for 9 mins

11. Release the valve and serve

MEAL PREP TIPS & TRICKS

I   An Instant Pot is another kitchen appliance not everyone has. If you have any type of pressure ccoker, by all means, give it a whirl, just keep your eye on it. Alternatively, swap the meal for something else.

DAY 13

Breakfast*: Egg and Hash

Serves 3 | kCal: 248 | Carbs: 5.77g | Fat: 18.14g | Prot: 12.57g

INGREDIENTS

- 5oz / 142gr of dried zucchini
- 6oz / 170gr of cauliflower, chopped
- ½ medium red bell pepper, diced
- 1 tablespoon / 15gr coconut oil, melted
- 1 teaspoon / 5gr paprika
- 1 teaspoon / 5gr onion powder
- ¼ cup / 85gr garlic powder
- ¼ cup / 85gr Mexican blend cheese, grated
- ½ medium avocado, sliced
- 3 large eggs
- 3 tablespoons / 42gr of cotija cheese
- 2 teaspoons / 10gr Tajin seasoning

DIRECTIONS

1. Preheat the oven to 400°F / 205°C
2. Line a baking tray with foil
3. Spread the zucchini, cauliflower, and pepper evenly and drizzle with the coconut oil
4. Sprinkle onion powder, garlic powder, and paprika and toss to coat everything evenly
5. Spread into a layer again
6. Bake for 10 – 15 mins until the vegetables start to brown
7. Remove the tray from the oven and sprinkle the Mexican cheese over the top of the veg
8. Arrange the avocado slices among the veg and crack the eggs into available spaces
9. Bake for another 10 mins until the eggs are done
10. Garnish with the cotija cheese and Tajin seasoning and serve

Lunch: Veggie Zucchini (See page 53)

Dinner: Chicken Roulade (See page 61)

MEAL PREP TIPS & TRICKS

I Seasonings and cheeses feature a lot in keto. When you shop, buy the ones you know you enjoy and stock up on them. Don't feel pressured to using the ones in the recipes. Enjoying your food is the way to stay on your diet.

DAY 14

Breakfast: Scrambled No-Eggs (See page 37)

Lunch*: Bacon Salad

Serves 2 | kCal: 328.55 | Carbs: 6.23g | Fat: 27.85g | Prot: 13.5g

INGREDIENTS

- 4 bacon slices
- 2 cup / 134gr kale
- ¼ cup / 35gr sweet onion
- ½ cup / 60gr raw walnuts

- 2 teaspoons / 6gr erythritol
- ½ teaspoon / 2.5ml maple syrup
- 1 tablespoon / 15ml lemon juice

DIRECTIONS

1. Cook the baconas you like it, plate and allow to cool
2. Cook the walnuts in the bacon grease on a medium heat, coating well with the grease
3. Chop the kale stems off and the leaves into bite sizes. Put into a salad bowl
4. Dice the onion
5. Sprinkle the erythritol and syrup over thecooking walnuts and coat evenly
6. Add the onion and sauté until soft and the walnuts have caramelized
7. Remove the pan from the heat and drizzle lemon juice over the walnuts
8. Cut the bacon into smaller pieces
9. Put the walnut mixture over the kale and toss to coat
10. Sprinkle the bacon over the top and serve

Dinner: Chicken Chili (See page 67)

MEAL PREP TIPS & TRICKS

| Don't like kale? Swap it for some lettuce.

DISCLAIMER

Printed in Great Britain
by Amazon